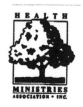

FAITH COMMUNITY NURSING:
SCOPE AND STANDARDS
OF PRACTICE

AMERICAN NURSES ASSOCIATION
SILVER SPRING, MD
2005

Library of Congress Cataloging-in-Publication data

Health Ministries Association.
  Faith community nursing : scope and standards of practice / Health
Ministries Association.
    p. ; cm.
  Includes bibliographical references and index.
  ISBN-13: 978-1-55810-228-6
  ISBN-10: 1-55810-228-0
  1. Parish nursing—Standards—United States. 2. Community health
nursing—Standards—United States. I. American Nurses Association.
II. Title.
  [DNLM: 1. Community Health Nursing—standards. 2. Spirituality.
3. Cultural Diversity. 4. Nursing Process—standards. 5. Religion.
WY 87 H434f 2005]
  RT120.P37H43 2005
  610.73'43—dc22   2005015923

The American Nurses Association (ANA) is a national professional association. This ANA publication—*Faith Community Nursing: Scope and Standards of Practice*—reflects the thinking of the nursing profession on various issues and should be reviewed in conjunction with state board of nursing policies and practices. State law, rules, and regulations govern the practice of nursing, while *Faith Community Nursing: Scope and Standards of Practice* guides nurses in the application of their professional skills and responsibilities.

Health Ministries Association (HMA), a non-profit organization, is a support network for people of faith who promote whole-person health through faith groups in the communities they serve. By providing information, guidelines, and resources, HMA assists and encourages individuals, called health ministers, as they develop whole-person health programs, utilize community resources, and educate others on the interdependent health of body, mind and spirit.

Published by nursesbooks.org
The Publishing Program of ANA

American Nurses Association
8515 Georgia Avenue, Suite 400
Silver Spring, MD 20910-3492
1-800-274-4ANA
http://www.nursesbooks.org/

ANA is the only full-service professional organization representing the nation's 2.7 million Registered Nurses through its 54 constituent member associations. ANA advances the nursing profession by fostering high standards of nursing practice, promoting the economic and general welfare of nurses in the workplace, projecting a positive and realistic view of nursing, and lobbying the Congress and regulatory agencies on healthcare issues affecting nurses and the public.

ISBN 978-1-55810-228-6   05SSFC   5M   01/06R

First printing June 2005.   Second printing January 2006.

ACKNOWLEDGMENTS

Work Group Members
Peggy S. Matteson, PhD, RN, FCN, *Chair*
Rev. Sheryl S. Cross, MSN, MDiv, RN, FCN
Dianne Foglesong, MSN, RN, FCN
Amy Hickman, BS, RN,
Lynne Roy, MSN, RN, FCN
Nancy L. Rago Durbin, MA, MS, RNC, FCN
Roberta Schweitzer, PhD, RN, FCN
Sonja Simpson, MSN, RN, HNC, FCN
Sybil D. Smith, PhD, RN, FCN
Susan L. Ward PhD, RN, FCN

ANA Staff
Carol Bickford, PhD, RN, BC – Content editor
Yvonne Humes, MSA – Project coordinator
Winifred Carson, JD – Legal counsel

CONTENTS

INTRODUCTION

There have been dramatic changes in health care and the profession of nursing during the past decade. *Nursing: Scope and Standards of Practice* (ANA 2004) provided the framework and direction for review and revision of this scope and standards of practice. The purpose of this document is to describe the specialty practice of faith community nursing and to provide faith community nurses, the nursing profession, other healthcare providers, spiritual leaders, employers, insurers, and their patients with an understanding of the unique scope of knowledge and the standards of care and professional performance expected of a faith community nurse (FCN).

Function of the Scope of Practice Statement of Faith Community Nursing

The scope of practice statement describes the *who, what, where, when, why,* and *how* of the practice of faith community nursing. The answers to these questions provide a complete picture of the practice, its boundaries, and its membership.

Nursing: Scope and Standards of Practice (ANA 2004*)* applies to all professional registered nurses engaged in practice, regardless of specialty, practice setting, or educational preparation. With *Code of Ethics for Nurses with Interpretive Statements* (ANA 2001*)* and *Nursing's Social Policy Statement* (ANA 2003), it forms the foundation of practice for all registered nurses. The scope of faith community nursing practice is specific to this specialty, but builds on the scope of care expected of all registered nurses.

Function of the Standards of Faith Community Nursing

"Standards are authoritative statements by which the nursing profession describes the responsibilities for which its practitioners are accountable. Consequently, standards reflect the values and priorities of the profession. Standards provide direction for professional nursing practice and a framework for evaluation of this practice. Written in measurable terms, these standards define the nursing profession's accountability to the public and the outcomes for which registered nurses are responsible" (ANA 2004, 1). The standards of faith community nursing practice are specific to this specialty, but build on the standards of care expected of all registered nurses.

Development of *Faith Community Nursing: Scope and Standards of Practice*

As the professional organization for all registered nurses, the American Nurses Association (ANA) has assumed the responsibility for developing generic scope and standards that apply to the practice of all professional nurses. *Nursing: Scope and Standards of Practice* (ANA 2004) describes what nursing is, what nurses do, and the responsibilities for which they are accountable.

Health Ministries Association (HMA), the professional membership organization for nurses in this specialty, and ANA collaborated in the development and publication of *Scope and Standards of Parish Nursing Practice* in 1998. With the publication of the new Foundation of Nursing documents, all specialty scope and standards are now being revised. For continuity and consistency, *Nursing: Scope and Standards of Practice* (ANA 2004) was used as the template when developing this document.

During 2003 and early 2004, HMA requested volunteers to serve on a working group to review and revise the scope and standards. Ten practicing nurses representing different parts of the country and various roles in this specialty practice convened and started work in February 2004. In August a draft was posted on the HMA web site for six weeks of public review. Hard copies of the document were also distributed on request. More than 200 responses were received and carefully considered. As a result, this document provides a national perspective on the current practice of this evolving specialty of faith community nursing.

Summary

These standards and scope of practice for faith community nursing reflect the commitment of Health Ministries Association, Inc., to work with American Nurses Association to promote understanding of faith community nursing as a specialized practice in the multidisciplinary practice arena of diverse faith communities. HMA is the national professional organization representing faith community nurses and others working in the expanding faith community arena.

As the diversity of participating faith communities expands in rural areas, towns, and cities, the difficulty in finding all-inclusive terminology to describe the beliefs and practices that have evolved from dissimilar traditions becomes more apparent. Terms used in this document indicate an effort to include all faith traditions, not to promote any one faith tradition.

Faith Community Nursing: Scope and Standards of Practice reflects current faith community nursing practice from a national perspective, the professional and ethical standards of the nursing profession, and the legal scope and standards of professional nursing practice. They are dynamic and subject to testing and change.

Standards of Faith Community Nursing Practice: Standards of Practice

Standard 1. Assessment
The faith community nurse collects comprehensive data pertinent to the patient's wholistic health or the situation.

Standard 2. Diagnosis
The faith community nurse analyzes the wholistic assessment data to determine the diagnoses or issues.

Standard 3. Outcomes Identification
The faith community nurse identifies expected outcomes for a plan individualized to the patient or the situation.

Standard 4. Planning
The faith community nurse develops a plan that prescribes strategies and alternatives to attain expected outcomes for individuals, groups, or the faith community as a whole.

Standard 5. Implementation
The faith community nurse implements the specified plan.

Standard 5a: Coordination of Care
The faith community nurse coordinates care delivery.

Standard 5b: Health Teaching and Health Promotion
The faith community nurse employs strategies to promote wholistic health, wellness, and a safe environment.

Standard 5c: Consultation
The faith community nurse provides consultation to facilitate understanding and influence the specified plan of care, enhance the abilities of others, and effect change.

Standard 5d: Prescriptive Authority and Treatment
(Optional for appropriately prepared APRN)
The advanced practice registered nurse, faith community nurse uses prescriptive authority, procedures, referrals, treatments, and therapies in accordance with state and federal laws and regulations.

Standard 6. Evaluation
The faith community nurse evaluates progress toward attainment of outcomes.

STANDARDS OF FAITH COMMUNITY NURSING PRACTICE: STANDARDS OF PROFESSIONAL PERFORMANCE

STANDARD 7. QUALITY OF PRACTICE

The faith community nurse systematically enhances the quality and effectiveness of faith community nursing practice.

STANDARD 8. EDUCATION

The faith community nurse attains knowledge and competency that reflects current nursing practice.

STANDARD 9. PROFESSIONAL PRACTICE EVALUATION

The faith community nurse evaluates one's own nursing practice in relation to professional practice standards and guidelines, relevant statutes, rules, and regulations.

STANDARD 10. COLLEGIALITY

The faith community nurse interacts with and contributes to the professional development of peers and colleagues.

STANDARD 11. COLLABORATION

The faith community nurse collaborates with the patient, spiritual leaders, members of the faith community, and others in the conduct of this specialized nursing practice.

STANDARD 12. ETHICS

The faith community nurse integrates ethical provisions in all areas of practice.

STANDARD 13. RESEARCH

The faith community nurse integrates research findings into practice.

STANDARD 14. RESOURCE UTILIZATION

The faith community nurse considers factors related to safety, effectiveness, cost, and impact on practice in the planning and delivery of nursing services.

STANDARD 15. LEADERSHIP

The faith community nurse provides leadership in the professional practice setting and the profession.

Scope of Faith Community Nursing Practice

Definition and Overview of Faith Community Nursing

> Faith community nursing is the specialized practice of professional nursing that focuses on the intentional care of the spirit as part of the process of promoting wholistic health and preventing or minimizing illness in a faith community.

The faith community nurse (FCN) is knowledgeable in two areas—professional nursing and spiritual care. As a member of the staff providing spiritual care in the faith community, the goal of an FCN is the protection, promotion, and optimization of health and abilities; prevention of illness and injury; and responding to suffering in the context of the values, beliefs, and practices of a faith community such as a church, congregation, parish, synagogue, temple, or mosque.

The FCN uses the nursing process to address the spiritual, physical, mental, and social health of the patient. The term *patient* may refer to the faith community as a whole, or groups, families, and individuals in the faith community. Residents from the vicinity of the faith community may also seek the services of the FCN.

With an intentional focus on spiritual health, the FCN primarily uses the nursing interventions of education, counseling, advocacy, referral, utilizing resources available to the faith community, and training and supervising volunteers from the faith community. As an actively licensed registered nurse, the FCN provides nursing care based on professional and legal expectations, education, professional experience, the needs of the patient population, and the position as defined in the faith community. The FCN collaborates with other nursing specialties such as community health, hospice, rehabilitation, home health, acute care, and critical care in other aspects of nursing care for the faith community and its members.

This document—in conjunction with *Nursing's Social Policy Statement* (ANA 2003); *Nursing: Scope and Standards of Practice* (ANA 2004); *Code of Ethics for Nurses with Interpretive Statements* (ANA 2001); and the laws, statutes, and regulations related to nursing practice for their state, commonwealth, or territory—delineates the professional responsibilities of an FCN.

Evolution of Faith Community Nursing

Nursing has its historical roots in the link between faith and healing in the ancient traditions of most major religions. This relationship evolved over time, influenced by cultural, political, social, and economic events. Religious groups founded hospitals to provide care to vulnerable populations such as the poor, immigrant, and homeless, and during the last century developed schools of nursing.

In 1979, Rev. Dr. Granger Westberg received grant funding to create Wholistic Health Centers in Christian congregations, staffed by a treatment/healing team comprised of a doctor, a nurse, a social worker, and a pastoral counselor. The nurses in these centers were referred to as "parish nurses." Since then various other faith communities have established programs of health and healing led by a registered nurse. The word "parish" in *parish nurse* is not acceptable in all faith traditions, so faith communities have created different titles for this specialized nursing role. To have one name inclusive of all faith traditions and to accurately label the location and focus of practice, the specialty practice described in this document is titled "faith community nursing." In a given setting, the faith community nurse may still be referred to as a *parish nurse, congregational nurse, health ministry nurse, crescent nurse,* or *health and wellness nurse.*

Westberg used the term "wholistic health" to define a whole or completely integrated approach to health and health care that integrates the physical and spiritual aspects of the whole person. The principles of wholistic health arose from the understanding that human beings strive for wholeness in relationship to their God, themselves, their families, and the society in which they live. Based on its historic meaning, then, *wholistic* is the preferred spelling when referring to the health care provided by faith community nurses.

Nurse-led programs within and beyond Judeo-Christian faith communities continue to grow and evolve. The common expectation across faith traditions is that the professional registered nurse functioning as an FCN possesses a depth of understanding of the faith community's traditions, as well as competence as a registered nurse using the nursing process so that the nursing care integrates care of the spirit with that of the body and mind.

Assumptions of Faith Community Nursing

These five assumptions underlie faith community nursing:

- Health and illness are human experiences.
- Health is the integration of the spiritual, physical, psychological, and social aspects of the patient promoting a sense of harmony with self, others, the environment, and a higher power.

- Health may be experienced in the presence of disease or injury.

- The presence of illness does not preclude health nor does optimal health preclude illness.

- Healing is the process of integrating the body, mind, and spirit to create wholeness, health, and a sense of well-being, even when the patient's illness is not cured.

Focusing on Spiritual Care in the Art of Nursing

Nurses have long observed that when illness or brokenness occurs, patients—whether individually or with their family or friends—may turn to their source of spiritual strength for reassurance, support, and healing. *Nursing: Scope and Standards of Practice* (ANA 2004) reaffirms that spiritual care is a part of all nursing practice. The primary focus of the FCN is the intentional care of the spirit, differentiating this specialty practice from the general practice of a registered nurse. Within this specialized knowledge base, each FCN will demonstrate competence on a continuum from novice to expert.

A variety of tools for spiritual assessment have been developed and tested for reliability and validity. These tools, varying from simple screening to in-depth assessments, are increasingly used in nursing practice. Since the use of spiritual assessment tools has not been generally taught to providers from other disciplines, the FCN may provide leadership to the staff in the selection and application of assessment tools.

After analyzing the assessment data, the FCN selects the nursing diagnoses to describe actual or potential needs of the patient, including spiritual needs. These diagnoses then provide the basis for nursing interventions to achieve the outcomes for which the nurse is accountable. Examples of nursing diagnoses accepted by the North American Nursing Diagnosis Association (NANDA) related specifically to spiritual care are Spiritual Distress, Risk for Spiritual Distress, and Readiness for Spiritual Well-being (NANDA 2005).

Treatment may or may not cure an affliction. However, it is still possible through care of the spirit for a person to be healed even if a cure—physical restoration—does not occur. A patient may be dying from cancer, but if a broken relationship between family members has been reconciled or the patient is at peace with the circumstances, this may be considered healing.

Assault, betrayal, accident, or death of a member can affect an entire faith community. Members of all ages may manifest anger, grief, anxiety, fear, and spiritual or physical pain in varying degrees. An FCN's response to such an event is complex. Beyond identifying and meeting the needs of individuals and families, the FCN treats the whole faith community as a patient. Assessment focuses on identifying the educational and supportive needs of the whole faith community. Interventions occur at three different levels: community, family or group, and individual.

From a less dramatic but equally important perspective, the FCN will address a variety of issues that threaten the wholistic health of participants in the faith community:

- Individuals or families may lack food, shelter, transportation, income, or health care.

- Victims of domestic violence or other forms of abuse may seek solace or sanctuary.

- Adult children of aging parents may seek guidance in talking with or determining the appropriate living situation for a parent, and ongoing assistance from the faith community.

To respond to these and other situations wholistically, an FCN draws on professional skills that integrate spiritual care and nursing care, and the resources of individuals and groups both within and beyond the faith community to provide a wholistic response. Some patients will require support of basic needs so that they have the time and space to reflect on spiritual issues; for others, spiritual care will be the direct response.

The form that spiritual care takes will depend upon the beliefs and practices of the faith community; the desire of the faith community, the group, or the individual; the skills of the faith community nurse; and the collaboration of other staff members and volunteers.

Educational Preparation for Faith Community Nursing

The faith community nurse bridges two disciplines and thus must be prepared in and responsible to both. This document provides a complete picture of the specialty practice and its boundaries and membership from the perspective of the nursing profession; each faith group may provide additional stipulations and requirements. There are designations in the specialty that indicate the level of education achieved.

Appropriate and effective practice as an FCN requires the ability to integrate current nursing, behavioral, environmental, and spiritual knowledge with the unique spiritual beliefs and practices of the faith community into a program of wholistic nursing care. This is necessary no matter what level of education the nurse has achieved. With education, mentoring, and a collaborative practice site, an FCN may progress from novice to expert in this specialty practice.

Faith Community Nurse

The preferred minimum preparation for a registered nurse or advanced practice registered nurse entering the specialty of faith community nursing includes:

- A baccalaureate or higher degree in nursing with academic preparation in community nursing,
- Experience as a registered nurse using the nursing process,
- Knowledge of the healthcare assets of the community,
- Specialized knowledge of the spiritual beliefs and practices of the faith community, and
- Specialized knowledge and skills to enable implementation of *Faith Community Nursing: Scope and Standards of Practice.*

Currently, the education of all nursing students preparing for the national examination for RN licensure includes basic content on spiritual care. In addition, an increasing number of undergraduate students during their community health courses participate in clinical experiences with faith community nurses. However, because of the intentional focus on spiritual care by the faith community nurse, this educational exposure is not adequate preparation for assuming the specialty role of an FCN.

A registered nurse may prepare for the specialty of faith community nursing in one of several ways. Educational offerings range from continuing education programs with extensive contact hours to baccalaureate and graduate level nursing courses. Some colleges that specialize in religious education also offer relevant courses or programs of study. Collaboration between disciplines has also led to the offering of dual master's degrees in nursing and theology or health ministry. Registered nurses may also participate in online education with or without academic credit. Faith communities understand, support, and often fund continuing education of FCNs to enhance their ability to provide spiritual care, knowing that this directly benefits their own programs.

Specialty certification programs generally require psychometrically sound and legally defensible certification examinations. These are possible only with sufficient applicants and adequate financial resources. At this time, specialty certification in faith community nursing is not available. Because faith community nurses work in churches, synagogues, temples, mosques, and other faith community settings and not in healthcare facilities, certification currently has little bearing on the decision of a committee or board in a faith community to engage the professional services of an FCN. Other models for specialty certification, such as professional portfolios, are being explored.

Advanced Practice Registered Nurse

Increasing numbers of advanced practice registered nurses (APRNs: nurse practitioners and clinical nurse specialists) are acquiring the additional specialized education that prepares them for practice as a faith community nurse. By definition, an advanced practice registered nurse has a master's or doctoral degree that prepares the nurse to be a clinical expert in evidence-based nursing practice. An APRN, FCN has earned the designation as either a clinical nurse specialist or a nurse practitioner, and has also prepared for the role of an FCN. The APRN, FCN integrates theoretical and evidence-based knowledge from graduate nursing education with the specialized education of an FCN regarding the structure, spiritual beliefs, and practices of the faith group. These advanced practice nurses are held to a higher standard of expertise when providing nursing care.

The APRN, FCN designs, implements, and evaluates both population-specific and patient-specific programs of wholistic care for the faith community. An APRN, FCN provides leadership in advancing this specialty nursing practice to achieve quality and cost-effective wholistic patient outcomes, and leads multidisciplinary groups in designing and implementing innovative alternative solutions to problems and patient issues essential to spiritual health and well-being.

In addition to providing nursing care, the APRN, FCN influences nursing care outcomes by serving as an advocate, consultant, or researcher in the specialty area; providing expert consultation for spiritual leaders and other healthcare providers; and by identifying and facilitating improvements in wholistic health care.

Laws, regulations, and rules concerning certification as an advanced practice nurse are issued by state licensing or regulatory boards, and vary among states. Each FCN seeking to attain the APRN designation must meet the requirements of the jurisdiction of practice as well as the standards of practice set forth in this document.

Additional Designations

National leaders of faith groups that recognize the importance of integrating this specialty nursing practice into faith communities have developed mechanisms for mentoring and providing informal and formal education in concepts of spiritual beliefs, practices, and rituals. When such facilities are available within the faith group, the FCN may work with the leadership of the faith community to meet the educational and practice requirements to earn formal designation as a spiritual leader.

Faith groups have different ways of designating or titling individuals who have attained an advanced level of preparation and often undergone examination to determine fitness for providing spiritual care. The FCN who achieves the requirements defined by the faith group in which they are practicing may then be given a title by the faith community indicating their achievement. Examples of such titles are *Deacon*, *Minister of Health*, or *Pastoral Associate*. Titles such as these have a specialized meaning within the faith community served.

Settings for Practice in Faith Community Nursing

An FCN serves as a member of the multidisciplinary staff of a faith community, providing care to the faith community as a whole as well as to member groups and individuals. The FCN is the sole healthcare provider responsible for practice in this non-healthcare setting, although others from the faith community assist the FCN.

Most encounters with patients are initiated within the buildings and programs of the faith community. Participants in the various activities of the faith community, such as worship, education, special interest or support groups, programs for spiritual growth or renewal, and support services such as soup kitchens, may seek the services of the FCN.

A community of faith may be composed of people of all ages. The members may also offer a range of physical, emotional, and cognitive development. When an individual, family, group, or the faith community as a whole experiences or desires a change in their level of physical, mental, social, environmental, or spiritual well-being, or when maintaining their current level of well-being requires nursing action, an FCN collaborates with them to develop a plan of care that incorporates communal and individual spiritual beliefs and practices.

The FCN monitors environmental and safety issues of the facilities and chooses appropriate responses in collaboration with the leadership of the faith community. The FCN also manages physical and mental health issues, including the high levels of stress of spiritual leaders, other staff members, or faith community volunteers, with interventions that encompass spiritual support, health promotion, illness prevention, and disease management.

The needs and desires of individual members of the faith community may require that the FCN visit members in the hospital or a hospice, in private homes or residential facilities, or accompany patients as they use health services in the community. During these encounters the FCN may also intervene with spiritual care and provide a supportive, healing presence for both the patient and loved ones.

The size, concerns, and expectations of the faith community will determine the expected role of an FCN. As a staff member, the FCN is most often supported and guided by a committee of faith community members and assisted by lay volunteers. With education and supervision provided by the FCN, these volunteers may assume tasks that family members would do for each other if they were available. This type of supportive team, led by the FCN, can increase safety and comfort during hospital discharge transitions and provide patients with comprehensive support once home, helping them to recuperate more easily or to achieve peace before death.

Continued Commitment to the Profession

The specialty practice of faith community nursing is relatively new, and requires that each FCN educate other healthcare providers and the general public concerning the benefits of this nursing care. An faith community nurse may participate with colleagues in the community, such as an FNC group or a clergy association, to develop collaborative efforts throughout the community.

The FCN commits to lifelong learning in both nursing and the beliefs and practices of the faith community. There are numerous opportunities for personal and professional growth both in and beyond the community. Major denominations support both programs and professional development. The professional organization for faith community nurses, the Health Ministries Association, provides opportunities for networking and ongoing education both in the specialty as well as with other disciplines. A variety of educational institutions and resource centers are also available around the country or online.

While the FCN may be the only healthcare provider in the faith community, the best practice cannot be provided in isolation. Personal and professional support, education opportunities, and resources are available. Accessing these will improve both the care provided to the faith community and the progress of the specialty.

Research

Research conducted at the National Institutes of Health and academic institutions has established a relationship between spiritual practices and health, thereby expanding the knowledge base for the specialty of faith community nursing. Findings from a variety of non-nursing disciplines provide understanding of the strong connection between spiritual well-being, participation in religious practices, and wholistic health. Involvement in a faith community provides health benefits through social support, a social identity, and a sense of power beyond one's self. Religious and spiritual practices such as meditation, prayer, and touch are reported to lengthen life, improve the quality of life, and improve health outcomes by enhancing psychological, physical, and spiritual well-being. Research reports may be found in the nursing literature and publications of other health professionals, as well as the professional literature focused on health ministry, chaplaincy, theology, spirituality, spiritual care, and pastoral care.

Research by faith community nurses to evaluate the benefits of this specialty practice is slowly emerging. Funding would enhance efforts to establish programs of collaborative research between practicing faith community nurses and nurse researchers that could validate and promote the wholistic health benefits of this nursing specialty in the multidisciplinary environment. Confirmation of positive outcomes would be a major influence in funding further research and positions for faith community nurses.

Professional Trends and Issues

Since 1998, when faith community nursing was formally recognized as a specialty practice, there has been tremendous growth in both professional knowledge and the number of faith communities seeking such services. With this growth, several issues have become more apparent:

- *What to call nurse providers so that the title is understood across various faith groups.* This issue has been addressed with the adoption of an all-encompassing title for this specialty. Sensitivity to the desires of individual faith communities to maintain their own internal title has also been considered. Just as each community calls their spiritual leader by their own title, such as rabbi, pastor, minister, teacher, they may also call the FCN by the title they choose. However, selection of an internal title different than faith community nurse does not relieve that registered nurse from fulfilling the expectations set forth in this document.

- *Identifying the preparation needed for this evolving specialty practice.* This discussion is ongoing. When educational resources for this specialty were difficult to obtain, nurses had minimal opportunities. With the clarification of minimum standards and an increasing awareness by nurse educators and practicing nurses of the requirements for this specialty practice, both educational expectations and opportunities are increasing at all levels of nursing education.

- *Engaging other practice disciplines and faith communities in accepting this specialty nursing practice.* As the number and professional activities of faith community nurses increase, so too does the recognition of these specialists by other disciplines. Faith community nurses are vital partners in advancing the nation's health initiatives such as Healthy People 2010 to increase the quality and years of healthy life and eliminate health disparities. As members of faith communities experience the benefit of care from an FCN and share their experiences with others, the demand for these services will increase.

- *Creation of paid positions so that more professional nurses may choose to enter the specialty.* Financial compensation for providing faith community nursing services is a complex subject familiar to those who know the history of compensation in professional nursing. In this case, the issue is complicated by three major factors:
  - A lack of financial resources in many faith communities for an expansion of services,
  - A faith community's tradition of donating time and expertise to care for each other, and
  - Difficulty in obtaining objective data that demonstrates the positive health affects and benefits of faith community nursing so that external funding will be more available.

As with any complex issue, addressing this situation will be a multifaceted process. Some faith community nurses choose to provide care part- or full-time, at low financial compensation if any, as part of their gift to the faith community. Others provide care so that they may demonstrate the value of this specialty practice and collect data to support the hiring of a faith community nurse for that community of faith. Some nurses, taking a broader perspective, work within faith community organizations to increase recognition of this specialty nursing practice as a form of spiritual leadership worthy of financial support. Still others are encouraging healthcare organizations and facilities to provide financial support of an FCN in faith communities. Given the varied dynamics of individual communities of faith, there is no one solution.

This document delineates the professional expectations associated with this specialty practice. When it is considered in conjunction with *Nursing's Social Policy Statement* (ANA 2003), *Nursing: Scope and Standards of Practice* (ANA 2004), and *Code of Ethics for Nurses with Interpretive Statements* (ANA 2001), the professional nurse receives clear guidance in the requirements for preparation and practice that best serve the public's health and the nursing profession.

STANDARDS OF FAITH COMMUNITY NURSING PRACTICE
STANDARDS OF PRACTICE

STANDARD 1. ASSESSMENT

The faith community nurse collects comprehensive data pertinent to the patient's wholistic health or the situation.

Measurement Criteria:

The faith community nurse:

- Prioritizes data collection activities based on the patient's immediate condition, or the anticipated needs of the patient or situation.
- Collects wholistic data in a systematic and ongoing process, with a particular emphasis on spiritual beliefs and practices.
- Involves the patient, family, group, spiritual leader, other healthcare providers, and others, as appropriate, in wholistic data collection.
- Uses appropriate evidence-based assessment techniques and instruments in collecting pertinent data as a basis for wholistic care.
- Uses analytical models and problem-solving tools.
- Synthesizes available data, information, and knowledge relevant to the situation to identify patterns and variances in individuals, families, groups, or the faith community as a whole.
- Documents and stores relevant data in a retrievable format that is both confidential and secure.

Additional Measurement Criteria for the Advanced Practice Registered Nurse, Faith Community Nurse:

The advanced practice registered nurse, faith community nurse:

- Interprets results from diagnostic tests relevant to the wholistic assessment of the patient's current status.

STANDARD 2. DIAGNOSIS

The faith community nurse analyzes the wholistic assessment data to determine the diagnoses or issues.

Measurement Criteria:

The faith community nurse:

- Derives the diagnoses or issues based on wholistic assessment data.
- Identifies strengths that enhance health and spiritual well-being.
- Identifies actual, perceived, or potential threats to health and spiritual well-being.
- Validates the diagnoses or issues with the patient, family, spiritual leader, and other healthcare providers, when possible and appropriate.
- Documents diagnoses in a manner that facilitates the determination of the expected outcomes and plan.

Additional Measurement Criteria for the Advanced Practice Registered Nurse, Faith Community Nurse:

The advanced practice registered nurse, faith community nurse:

- Systematically compares and contrasts assessment data with normal and abnormal variations and developmental events in formulating a differential diagnosis.
- Utilizes complex data and information obtained during interview, wholistic assessment, and diagnostic procedures in identifying diagnoses.
- Assists registered nurses in developing and maintaining competency in the diagnostic process.

Standard 3. Outcomes Identification

The faith community nurse identifies expected outcomes for a plan individualized to the patient or the situation.

Measurement Criteria:

The faith community nurse:

- Involves the patient, spiritual leaders, and healthcare providers in formulating expected outcomes when possible and as appropriate.
- Derives culturally and spiritually appropriate expected outcomes from the identified diagnoses.
- Considers spiritual beliefs and practices, associated benefits, costs, risks, current scientific evidence, and clinical expertise when formulating expected outcomes.
- Defines expected outcomes in terms of the patient, patient values, faith beliefs and practices, ethical considerations, family perspectives, cultural practices, environment, or situation with such considerations as associated benefits, risks, and costs, and current scientific evidence.
- Develops expected outcomes that focus on patients attaining, maintaining, or regaining health or healing, with a particular emphasis on patient-identified spiritual well-being.
- Identifies expected outcomes that incorporate spiritual beliefs and practices with current scientific evidence and are achievable through implementation of evidence-based practices.
- Includes a realistic time estimate for attainment of expected outcomes.
- Develops in a collaborative process expected outcomes that provide direction for continuity of care.
- Modifies expected outcomes based on changes in the desires of the patient, the status of the patient, or evaluation of the situation.
- Documents expected outcomes as measurable goals.

Continued ▶

Additional Measurement Criteria for the Advanced Practice Registered Nurse, Faith Community Nurse:

The advanced practice registered nurse, faith community nurse:

- Identifies expected outcomes that incorporate patient satisfaction with care and quality of life, cost and clinical effectiveness, and continuity and consistency between patient's spiritual beliefs and healthcare interventions.
- Supports the use of clinical and spiritual guidelines linked to positive patient outcomes of wholistic health and healing.

STANDARD 4. PLANNING

The faith community nurse develops a plan that prescribes strategies and alternatives to attain expected outcomes for individuals, groups, or the faith community as a whole.

Measurement Criteria:

The faith community nurse:

- Develops an individualized plan considering patient characteristics, spiritual beliefs and practices, and the situation.
- Develops the plan in conjunction with the patient, spiritual leaders, and others, as appropriate.
- Includes strategies in the plan that address each of the identified diagnoses or issues, which may include strategies for promotion and restoration of health, spiritual enhancement, and prevention of illness, injury, and disease.
- Integrates current trends and research affecting care in the planning process.
- Defines the plan to reflect current statutes, rules, regulations, and standards.
- Considers the economic impact of the plan and how the faith community and local community resources might be of assistance.
- Establishes the priorities in the plan with the patient, and others, as appropriate.
- Participates in the design and development of multidisciplinary and interdisciplinary processes to address the situation or issue.
- Incorporates an implementation pathway or realistic timeline in the plan.
- Provides for continuity of care and appropriate communication in the plan.
- Uses recognized terminology or standardized language to document the plan.
- Communicates the plan, with the consent of the patient, to others involved in providing care.

Continued ▶

- Supports the integration of the resources of the faith community to enhance and complete the patient's decision-making processes.
- Utilizes the plan to provide direction to other members of the healthcare team.
- Contributes to the development and continuous improvement of the organizational systems of the faith community that support the planning process.

Additional Measurement Criteria for the Advanced Practice Registered Nurse, Faith Community Nurse:

The advanced practice registered nurse, faith community nurse:

- Identifies assessment, diagnostic strategies, and therapeutic interventions in the plan that reflect current evidence, including data, research, literature, and expert nursing knowledge to enhance wholistic health.
- Selects or designs strategies to meet the multifaceted wholistic needs of complex patients.
- Includes the synthesis of patients' values and spiritual beliefs regarding nursing and medical therapies in the plan.

STANDARD 5. IMPLEMENTATION

The faith community nurse implements the specified plan.

Measurement Criteria:

The faith community nurse:

- Collaborates with the patient and support system to implement the plan in a safe and timely manner.

- Collaborates with and empowers patients to enhance their spiritual well-being and healthy behaviors, reduce the occurrence of illness, modify health risk behaviors, and adapt to chronic changes in health status.

- Documents implementation and any modifications, including changes or omissions, of the specified plan.

- Utilizes evidence-based interventions and treatments specific to the diagnosis or issue.

- Utilizes resources and systems in the faith community and the community in which it is located to implement the plan.

- Collaborates with spiritual leaders, faith community volunteers, caregivers, nursing colleagues, and others to implement the plan.

- Fosters organizational systems and programs in the faith community that support implementation of the plan.

Additional Measurement Criteria for the Advanced Practice Registered Nurse, Faith Community Nurse:

The advanced practice registered nurse, faith community nurse:

- Develops and utilizes systems in the faith community and other community resources when necessary to implement the plan.

- Supports the development of multidisciplinary collaboration to implement the plan.

- Incorporates new knowledge and strategies to initiate change in faith community nursing care practices if desired outcomes are not achieved.

STANDARD 5A: COORDINATION OF CARE

The faith community nurse coordinates care delivery.

Measurement Criteria:

The faith community nurse:

- Coordinates implementation of the plan of care.
- Advocates for the patient's desired plan of care with other professionals and healthcare agencies.
- Documents the coordination of care in a secure and retrievable format.

Additional Measurement Criteria for the Advanced Practice Registered Nurse, Faith Community Nurse:

The advanced practice registered nurse, faith community nurse:

- Provides leadership in the coordination of multidisciplinary health care for integrated delivery of patient care services for members of a faith community.
- Synthesizes data and information to prescribe necessary system and community support measures, including environmental modifications, spiritual support, and faith-based interventions.
- Coordinates system and community resources that enhance delivery of care across continuums.

STANDARD 5B: HEALTH TEACHING AND HEALTH PROMOTION

The faith community nurse employs strategies to promote wholistic health, wellness, and a safe environment.

Measurement Criteria:

The faith community nurse:

- Teaches activities that strengthen the body–mind–spirit connection such as meditation, prayer, and guided imagery.

- Facilitates educational programs for individuals or groups that address such topics as spiritual practices for health and healing, healthy lifestyles, risk-reducing behaviors, developmental needs, activities of daily living, and self-care.

- Uses health promotion and health teaching methods appropriate to the situation, the faith community, and the patient's spiritual beliefs and practices, developmental level, learning needs, readiness, ability to learn, language or communication preference, and culture.

- Evaluates health information resources for use in faith community nursing for accuracy, readability, and comprehensibility by patients, and compatibility with patients' spiritual beliefs and practices.

- Seeks ongoing opportunities for feedback and evaluation of the effectiveness of the strategies used.

Additional Measurement Criteria for the Advanced Practice Registered Nurse, Faith Community Nurse:

The advanced practice registered nurse, faith community nurse:

- Synthesizes empirical evidence on spiritual practices, risk behaviors, learning theories, behavioral change theories, motivational theories, epidemiology, and other related theories and frameworks when designing wholistic health information and patient education.

- Designs health information and patient education appropriate to the patient's spiritual beliefs and practices, cultural values and beliefs, developmental level, learning needs, readiness to learn, and readiness to experience new spiritual practices.

- Evaluates health information resources, such as the Internet, for accuracy, readability, and comprehensibility to help patients access quality health information that is compatible with their spiritual beliefs and practices.

STANDARD 5C: CONSULTATION

The faith community nurse provides consultation to facilitate understanding and influence the specified plan of care, enhance the abilities of others, and effect change.

Measurement Criteria:

The faith community nurse:

- Synthesizes information on beliefs and practices of the faith community when providing consultation.
- Facilitates the effectiveness of a consultation by involving the patient in the decision-making process and negotiation of role responsibilities.

Additional Measurement Criteria for the Advanced Practice Registered Nurse, Faith Community Nurse:

The advanced practice registered nurse, faith community nurse:

- Synthesizes spiritual practices, organizational structure and beliefs of the faith group, clinical data, theoretical frameworks, and evidence when providing consultation.
- Facilitates the effectiveness of a consultation by involving the patient or their designee in decision-making and negotiating role responsibilities for each member of the faith community team.

STANDARD 5D: PRESCRIPTIVE AUTHORITY AND TREATMENT
(Optional for appropriately prepared APRN)

The advanced practice registered nurse, faith community nurse uses prescriptive authority, procedures, referrals, treatments, and therapies in accordance with state and federal laws and regulations.

Measurement Criteria for the Advanced Practice Registered Nurse, Faith Community Nurse:

The advanced practice registered nurse, faith community nurse:

- Prescribes evidence-based treatments, therapies, and procedures, considering the patient's comprehensive healthcare needs and their spiritual needs, beliefs, and practices.

- Prescribes therapies, including those that strengthen the body–mind–spirit connection such as meditation, prayer, guided imagery, and various rituals of worship.

- Prescribes pharmacological agents based on a current knowledge of pharmacology and physiology.

- Prescribes specific pharmacological agents and treatments based on clinical indicators, the patient's status and needs, and the results of diagnostic assessments and laboratory tests.

- Evaluates therapeutic and potential adverse effects of pharmacological and non-pharmacological treatments.

- Provides patients with information about intended effects and potential adverse effects of proposed prescriptive therapies.

- Provides information about costs, and complementary and alternative treatments and procedures, as appropriate.

STANDARD 6. EVALUATION

The faith community nurse evaluates progress toward attainment of outcomes.

Measurement Criteria:

The faith community nurse:

- Conducts a wholistic, systematic, ongoing, and criterion-based evaluation of the outcomes in relation to the structures and processes described by the plan and the indicated timeline.

- Includes the patient and others involved in the care or situation in the evaluative process.

- Evaluates the effectiveness of the planned strategies in relation to patient responses and attainment of expected outcomes.

- Documents the results of the evaluation, including results from the faith or spiritual realm.

- Uses ongoing assessment data to revise the diagnoses, the outcomes, the plan, and the implementation as needed.

- Disseminates the results to the patient and others involved in the care or situation, as appropriate, in accordance with state and federal laws and regulations.

- Uses the results of the evaluation analyses to make or recommend process or program changes in the faith community, as appropriate, to improve the provision and outcomes of care.

Additional Measurement Criteria for the Advanced Practice Registered Nurse, Faith Community Nurse:

The advanced practice registered nurse, faith community nurse:

- Evaluates the accuracy of the diagnosis and effectiveness of the interventions in relation to the patient's attainment of expected outcomes.

- Synthesizes the results of the evaluation analyses to determine the impact of the plan on the affected patients, families, groups, faith communities and institutions, collegial networks, organizations, and geopolitical communities.

- Uses the results of the evaluation analyses to increase awareness beyond the individual faith community of the wholistic health benefits and spiritual care provided through faith community nursing.

Standards of Professional Performance

Standard 7. Quality of Practice

The faith community nurse systematically enhances the quality and effectiveness of faith community nursing practice.

Measurement Criteria:

The faith community nurse:

- Obtains and maintains designation and recognition as a spiritual care provider in a faith community.

- Demonstrates quality by documenting the application of the nursing process in a responsible, accountable, and ethical manner.

- Uses the results of quality improvement activities to initiate changes in the practice of faith community nursing and in the interaction between a faith community and the healthcare delivery system.

- Uses creativity and innovation in faith community nursing practice to improve care delivery.

- Incorporates new knowledge to initiate changes in faith community nursing practice if desired outcomes are not achieved.

- Participates in quality improvement activities for faith community nursing. Such activities may include:

  - Identifying aspects of practice important for quality monitoring.
  - Using indicators developed to monitor quality and effectiveness.
  - Collecting data to monitor quality and effectiveness.
  - Analyzing quality data to identify opportunities for improving practice.
  - Formulating recommendations to improve practice or outcomes.
  - Implementing activities to enhance the quality of practice.
  - Developing, implementing, and evaluating policies, procedures, and guidelines.
  - Participating on interdisciplinary teams to evaluate clinical care or health services.
  - Participating in efforts to minimize costs and unnecessary duplication.
  - Analyzing factors related to safety, satisfaction, effectiveness, and cost–benefit options.

Continued ▶

- Analyzing leadership and organizational systems in the faith community for barriers.
- Implementing processes to remove or decrease barriers in the leadership and organizational structure of the faith community.

Additional Measurement Criteria for the Advanced Practice Registered Nurse, Faith Community Nurse:

The advanced practice registered nurse, faith community nurse:

- Obtains and maintains official designation and recognition in the faith community as a spiritual care leader, if available.
- Designs quality improvement initiatives.
- Implements initiatives to evaluate the need for change.
- Develops indicators to monitor quality and effectiveness of faith community nursing practice.
- Evaluates the practice environment and quality of nursing care rendered in relation to existing evidence, identifying opportunities for the generation and use of research.

STANDARD 8. EDUCATION

The faith community nurse attains knowledge and competency that reflects current nursing practice.

Measurement Criteria:

The faith community nurse:

- Participates in ongoing educational activities related to spiritual care, professional nursing practice, and related professional issues.

- Demonstrates a commitment to lifelong learning through self-reflection and inquiry to identify learning needs.

- Seeks learning experiences that reflect current practice in order to maintain knowledge, skills, and competence in all dimensions of faith community nursing.

- Acquires knowledge and skills appropriate to faith community nursing practice.

- Maintains professional records that provide evidence of competency and lifelong learning in the specialty.

- Seeks experiences and formal and independent learning activities to maintain and develop the necessary professional skills and knowledge to provide spiritual care.

- Uses current research findings and other evidence to expand knowledge and enhance role performance.

Additional Measurement Criteria for the Advanced Practice Registered Nurse, Faith Community Nurse:

The advanced practice registered nurse, faith community nurse:

- Uses current healthcare research findings and other evidence to expand clinical and professional knowledge in order to better combine two disciplines, nursing and spiritual care, into one practice role.

STANDARD 9. PROFESSIONAL PRACTICE EVALUATION

The faith community nurse evaluates one's own nursing practice in relation to professional practice standards and guidelines, relevant statutes, rules, and regulations.

Measurement Criteria:

The faith community nurse's practice reflects the application of knowledge of current practice standards, guidelines, statutes, rules, and regulations.

The faith community nurse:

- Provides age-appropriate care in a spiritually, culturally, and ethnically sensitive manner.

- Engages in self-evaluation of practice on a regular basis, identifying areas of strength as well as areas in which professional development would be beneficial.

- Obtains informal feedback regarding spiritual care and nursing practice from patients, peers, spiritual leaders, health committee members, faith community volunteers, professional colleagues, and others.

- Participates in systematic formal review, as appropriate.

- Takes action to achieve goals identified during the evaluation process.

- Provides rationales for practice beliefs, decisions, and actions as part of the informal and formal evaluation processes.

Additional Measurement Criteria for the Advanced Practice Registered Nurse, Faith Community Nurse:

The advanced practice registered nurse, faith community nurse:

- Engages in a formal process, seeking feedback regarding the integration of advanced nursing practice and spiritual care from patients, peers, professional colleagues, and others.

STANDARD 10. COLLEGIALITY

The faith community nurse interacts with and contributes to the professional development of peers and colleagues.

Measurement Criteria:

The faith community nurse:

- Shares knowledge and skills with peers and colleagues as evidenced by activities such as patient care conferences with spiritual leaders and other healthcare providers and presentations at formal or informal meetings.
- Provides peers with feedback regarding their practice and role performance.
- Interacts with peers and colleagues to enhance one's own professional faith community nursing practice, spiritual development, and role performance.
- Maintains compassionate and caring relationships with peers and colleagues.
- Contributes to an environment that is conducive to the education of colleagues concerning the relationship between spiritual care and wholistic health.
- Contributes to a supportive, healthy, spirit-filled work environment.
- Develops a plan for ongoing spiritual care and support of wholistic health of self and colleagues.
- Participates with colleagues to directly or indirectly advance wholistic health services and spiritual well-being in faith communities.
- Mentors other faith community nurses and colleagues as appropriate.

Additional Measurement Criteria for the Advanced Practice Registered Nurse, Faith Community Nurse:

The advanced practice registered nurse, faith community nurse:

- Models expert practice to interdisciplinary team members and healthcare consumers.
- Participates with interdisciplinary teams that contribute to role development of faith community nursing practice and faith community advanced practice nursing and wholistic health care.

STANDARD 11. COLLABORATION

The faith community nurse collaborates with the patient, spiritual leaders, members of the faith community, and others in the conduct of this specialized nursing practice.

Measurement Criteria:

The faith community nurse:

- Communicates with patient, family, groups, spiritual leaders, and other healthcare providers regarding the care that is needed and the faith community nurse's role in the provision of that care.

- Collaborates in creating a documented plan, focused on outcomes and decisions related to care and delivery of services, that indicates communication and coordination with the patient and others.

- Partners with others to enhance faith-based health care and ultimately care of the patient, through activities such as worship, prayer, education concerning spiritual practices, management of resources, program development, or research opportunities.

- Documents referrals, including provisions for continuity of care outside the faith community.

Additional Measurement Criteria for the Advanced Practice Registered Nurse, Faith Community Nurse:

The advanced practice registered nurse, faith community nurse:

- Partners with other disciplines to enhance faith-based patient care through interdisciplinary activities such as spiritual practices and worship, education, consultation, management, or research opportunities.

- Facilitates an interdisciplinary process with spiritual leaders and other professionals working within the faith community.

- Develops mechanisms to improve communication of plans of care, rationales for plan of care changes, and collaborative discussions to improve patient care.

Standard 12. Ethics

The faith community nurse integrates ethical provisions in all areas of practice.

Measurement Criteria:

The faith community nurse:

- Uses *Code of Ethics for Nurses with Interpretive Statements* (ANA 2001) to guide practice.
- Acknowledges and respects tenets of faith and spiritual belief system of a patient.
- Delivers care in a manner that preserves and protects patient autonomy, dignity, rights, and spiritual beliefs and practices.
- Maintains patient confidentiality within religious, legal, and regulatory parameters.
- Serves as a patient advocate assisting patients in developing skills for self-advocacy in support of their spiritual beliefs and practices.
- Maintains a therapeutic and professional patient–nurse relationship within appropriate professional role boundaries.
- Demonstrates a commitment to practicing self-care, growing spiritually, managing stress, and remaining connected both with a centered self and with others.
- Contributes to resolving ethical issues of patients, colleagues, or systems as evidenced in such activities as participating on ethics committees.
- Reports illegal, incompetent, or impaired practices.
- Participates on multidisciplinary and interdisciplinary teams that address ethical risks, benefits, and outcomes.

Additional Measurement Criteria for the Advanced Practice Registered Nurse, Faith Community Nurse:

The advanced practice registered nurse, faith community nurse:

- Informs the patient of the risks, benefits, and outcomes of healthcare regimens.
- Participates on multidisciplinary and interdisciplinary teams that address ethical risks, benefits, and outcomes of programs and decisions that affect health and healthcare delivery.

STANDARD 13. RESEARCH

The faith community nurse integrates research findings into practice.

Measurement Criteria:

The faith community nurse:

- Utilizes the best available evidence, including research findings, to guide practice decisions.

- Actively participates in research activities related to spirituality and health at the level appropriate to the faith community nurse's level of education and position. Such activities may include:

  - Identifying clinical and spiritual issues specific to nursing research.
  - Participating in data collection (surveys, pilot projects, formal studies).
  - Participating in a formal research committee or program.
  - Sharing research activities and findings with peers and others.
  - Conducting research.
  - Critically analyzing and interpreting research for application to practice in a faith community.
  - Using research findings in the development of policies, procedures, and standards of practice for wholistic patient care.
  - Incorporating research as a basis for learning.

Additional Measurement Criteria for the Advanced Practice Registered Nurse, Faith Community Nurse:

The advanced practice registered nurse, faith community nurse:

- Contributes to nursing knowledge by conducting or synthesizing research that discovers, examines, and evaluates knowledge, theories, criteria, and creative approaches to integrating spiritual care and nursing care in a faith community.

- Formally disseminates research findings through interdisciplinary activities such as presentations, publications, consultations, and journal clubs.

STANDARD 14. RESOURCE UTILIZATION

The faith community nurse considers factors related to safety, effectiveness, cost, and impact on practice in the planning and delivery of nursing services.

Measurement Criteria:

The faith community nurse:

- Evaluates factors such as safety, effectiveness, availability of other resources, cost and benefits, efficiencies, and impact on practice, when choosing between plans of care that would result in the same outcome.
- Assists the patient in identifying and securing appropriate and available resources to address health and spiritually related needs.
- Assigns or delegates tasks, based on the needs and condition of the patient, potential for harm, stability of the patient's condition, complexity of the task, and predictability of the outcome.
- Assists the patient in becoming an informed consumer about the options, costs, risks, and benefits of various interventions.
- Develops innovative solutions and applies strategies to obtain appropriate resources for faith community nursing care.

Additional Measurement Criteria for the Advanced Practice Registered Nurse, Faith Community Nurse:

The advanced practice registered nurse, faith community nurse:

- Utilizes organizational and community resources to formulate multidisciplinary and interdisciplinary plans of care.
- Develops innovative solutions and applies strategies to obtain appropriate resources for patient care problems that address effective resource utilization and maintenance of quality.
- Develops evaluation strategies to demonstrate cost-effectiveness, cost–benefit, and efficiency factors associated with faith community nursing practice.

STANDARD 15. LEADERSHIP

The faith community nurse provides leadership in the professional practice setting and the profession.

Measurement Criteria:

The faith community nurse:

- Engages in practice as a recognized member of the staff serving the faith community.

- Works to create and maintain healthy work environments in the local faith community.

- Displays the ability to define a clear vision, the associated goals, and a plan to implement and measure progress towards wholistic health through spiritual care.

- Demonstrates a commitment to continuous, lifelong learning and spiritual growth for self and others.

- Teaches others to succeed by mentoring and other strategies.

- Exhibits creativity and flexibility through times of change.

- Demonstrates energy, excitement, and a passion for quality, spirit-filled work.

- Willingly accepts mistakes by self and others, thereby creating a culture in which risk-taking is not only safe, but expected.

- Inspires loyalty by valuing people as the most precious asset in the faith community.

- Directs the coordination of care within the faith community, across settings, and among caregivers, including training and oversight of unlicensed volunteers in any assigned or delegated tasks.

- Serves in key roles in the faith community by participating on committees, councils, and administrative teams.

- Promotes advancement of faith community nursing and the profession of nursing through participation in professional organizations of nursing and clergy.

Additional Measurement Criteria for the Advanced Practice Registered Nurse, Faith Community Nurse:

The advanced practice registered nurse, faith community nurse:

- Works to influence decision-making bodies to recognize spiritual care as integral to improved patient care.
- Designs innovations to effect change in faith community nursing practice and outcomes.
- Provides direction to enhance the creation of multidisciplinary healthcare teams that include providers of spiritual care.
- Initiates revision of protocols or guidelines for outpatient care to reflect evidence-based faith community nursing practice, to reflect the benefit of care management by faith community nurses, or to address emerging problems.
- Promotes communication of information and advancement of faith community nursing through writing, publishing, and presentations for professional or lay audiences.
- Designs innovations to effect change in faith community nursing practice and improve the outcomes of wholistic health and healing.

Glossary

Advanced Practice Registered Nurse, Faith Community Nurse (APRN, FCN).
An Advanced Practice Registered Nurse, Faith Community Nurse (APRN, FCN) has earned designation as either a clinical nurse specialist or a nurse practitioner, and has also prepared for the role of an FCN. The APRN, FCN builds on the knowledge and skills of a faith community registered nurse by attaining and demonstrating a greater depth and breadth of knowledge, synthesis of data, increased complexity of skills, and interventions in the practice of faith community nursing. (*See also* Faith Community Nurse.)

Assessment. A systematic, dynamic process by which a faith community registered nurse, through interaction with the patient, family, groups, communities, populations, spiritual leaders, and healthcare providers, collects and analyzes data. In addition to spiritual assessment, the faith community registered nurse may include the following dimensions: physical, psychological, sociocultural, cognitive, functional abilities, developmental, economic, environment, and lifestyle.

Caregiver. A person who provides direct care for another, such as a child, dependent adult, the disabled, chronically ill, or spiritually distressed.

Code of ethics. A succinct list of provisions that makes explicit the primary goals, values, and obligations of the profession.

Continuity of care. An interdisciplinary process that includes patients, families, significant others, and appropriate members of a faith community in the development of a coordinated plan of care. This process facilitates the patient's transition between settings and healthcare providers, based on changing needs and available resources.

Criteria. Relevant, measurable indicators of the standards of practice and professional performance. Criteria are revised periodically to remain current with the evolving knowledge and practice of faith community nursing.

Data. Discrete entities that are described objectively without interpretation.

Diagnosis. A clinical judgment about the patient's response to actual, perceived, or potential health concerns or needs. The diagnosis provides the basis for determination of a plan to achieve desired outcomes, establish priorities, and develop a plan of action with the patient. Faith community registered nurses utilize nursing diagnoses or medical diagnoses depending on their education, clinical preparation, and legal authority.

Disease. A biological or psychosocial disorder of structure or function in a patient, especially one that produces specific signs or symptoms or that affects a specific part of the body, mind, or spirit.

Documentation. The recording of the assessment, plan of care, interventions, and evaluation of outcomes in a retrievable format that is both confidential and secure for the patient in order to facilitate continuity in meeting desired health outcomes.

Environment. The atmosphere, milieu, or conditions in which an individual lives, works, plays, or carries out their faith practices.

Evaluation. The process of determining the progress toward attainment of expected outcomes and the satisfaction of the patient with those outcomes, for the purpose of modifying the plan. Outcomes include the effectiveness of care, when addressing one's own practice.

Evidence-based practice. A process founded on the collection, interpretation, and integration of valid, important, and applicable patient-reported, clinician-observed, and research-derived evidence. The best available evidence, moderated by patient circumstances and preferences, is applied to improve the quality of clinical judgments.

Faith community. An organization of groups, families, and individuals who share common values, beliefs, religious doctrine, and faith practices that influence their lives, such as a church, synagogue, temple, or mosque, and that functions as a patient system, providing a setting for faith community nursing.

Faith Community Nurse (FCN). A registered professional nurse, actively licensed with the state, who serves as a member of the staff of a faith community. The FCN promotes health as wholeness of the faith community, its groups, families, and individual members, and the community it serves through the practice of nursing as defined by the nurse practice act in the jurisdiction in which the FCN practices and the standards of practice set forth in this document. (*See also* Advanced Practice Registered Nurse, Faith Community Nurse.)

Faith Community Nursing. The specialized practice of professional nursing that focuses on the intentional care of the spirit as part of the process of promoting wholistic health and preventing or minimizing illness in a faith community.

Family. Family of origin or significant others as identified by the patient. The patient may refer to some or all of the members of a faith community as part of their family.

Group. A number of people sharing something in common such as an interest, activity, or spiritual beliefs and practices.

Guidelines. Systematic statements that describe recommended actions based on available scientific evidence and expert opinion. Clinical guidelines describe a process of patient care management that has the potential of improving the quality of clinical and consumer decision-making.

Healing. The process of integrating the body, mind, and spirit to bring about wholeness, health, and a sense of spiritual well-being, although the patient's disease may not be cured.

Health. The experience of wholeness, salvation, or shalom. The integration of the spiritual, physical, psychological, and social aspects of the patient to create a sense of harmony with self, others, the environment, and a higher power. Health may be experienced in the presence or absence of disease or injury.

Healthcare providers. Individuals with special expertise who provide healthcare services or assistance to patients. They may include nurses, physicians, spiritual leaders, psychologists, social workers, nutritionists/dietitians, and various therapists.

Health ministry. The promotion of health and healing as part of the mission and service of a faith community to its members and the community it serves.

Health promotion. Activities and interventions that patients undertake to achieve desired health outcomes. Health promotion outcomes may be primary—the prevention of disease and injury; secondary—the early detection and appropriate intervention in illness or brokenness; or tertiary—the promotion of wholeness and sense of well-being when curing may not occur.

Illness. The subjective experience of discomfort, brokenness; the disintegration of body, mind, spirit; disharmony with others, the environment, or a higher power.

Implementation. The carrying out of a plan of action in a spiritual, caring relationship that provides the information, skills, motivation, spiritual or faith tradition rituals, and resources necessary to empower the patient to achieve desired health outcomes.

Interdisciplinary. Reliant on overlapping skills and knowledge of each team member and discipline, resulting in synergistic effects where outcomes are enhanced and more comprehensive than the simple aggregation of any team member's individual efforts.

Multidisciplinary. Reliant on each team member or discipline contributing discipline-specific skills.

Patient. Recipient of nursing practice; a human system (faith community, group, family, or individual) and its environment, viewed as an integrated whole for which the Faith Community Nurse provides professional services. The term *patient* is used to provide consistency and brevity, bearing in mind that other terms, such as *client, individual, family, groups, community,* or *population* might be better choices in some instances. When the patient is an individual, the focus is on the health state, problems, or needs of the individual. When the patient is a family or group, the focus is on the health of the unit as a whole or the reciprocal effects of the individual's health on the other members of the unit. When the patient is a community or population, the focus is on personal and environmental health and the health risks of the community or population.

Pastoral care. The practical expression of presence and guidance by a spiritual leader to support, nurture, or encourage the personal, spiritual, and social well-being of an individual or group in the faith community.

Peer review. A collegial, systematic, and periodic process by which Faith Community Nurses are held accountable for their practice and which foster the refinement of one's knowledge, skills, and decision-making.

Plan. A comprehensive outline of the components that need to be completed to attain mutually identified and expected patient outcomes.

Quality of care. The degree to which health services for patients, families, groups, communities, or populations increase the likelihood of desired outcomes, and are consistent with current professional knowledge.

Restorative practices. Nursing interventions that mitigate the impact of illness or disease.

Self-care. Actions a faith community, group, family, or individual take to attain desired wholistic health outcomes when they possess the requisite knowledge, skills, ability, resources, motivation, encouragement, and support.

Spiritual care. Interventions, individual or communal, that facilitate the ability to experience the integration of the body, mind, and spirit to achieve wholeness, health, and a sense of connection to self, others, and a higher power.

Spiritual leader. An individual recognized and authorized by a faith community, such as a clergyperson (pastor, priest, rabbi, shaman), chaplain, or lay minister, who guides and inspires others in the study and nurture of their spiritual beliefs and application of spiritual practices.

Standard. An authoritative statement defined and promoted by the profession that reflects the values held by the profession and specialized area of practice, and by which the quality of practice, service, or education can be evaluated.

Supportive practices. Nursing interventions that are oriented toward modification of relationships or the environment to support health.

Well-being. An individual's perception of their own wholistic health.

Wholistic. Based on an understanding that a patient is an interconnected unity and that physical, mental, social, environmental, and spiritual factors need to be included in any interventions. The whole system, whether referring to a human being or a faith community, is greater than the sum of its parts. The preferred term when referring to the type of care provided by a Faith Community Nurse.

REFERENCES

American Nurses Association. 2001. *Code of ethics for nurses with interpretive statements.* Washington, DC: Nursebooks.org.

————. 2003. *Nursing's social policy statement.* 2nd edition. Washington, DC: Nursebooks.org.

————. 2004. *Nursing: Scope and standards of practice.* Washington, DC: Nursebooks.org.

Health Ministries Association (HMA) and American Nurses Association (ANA). 1998. *Scope and standards of parish nursing practice.* Washington, DC: American Nurses Publishing.

North American Nursing Diagnosis Association (NANDA). 2005. *Nursing diagnoses: Definitions and classification 2005–*2006. Philadelphia: NANDA International.

APPENDIX A.
SCOPE AND STANDARDS OF PARISH NURSING PRACTICE (1998)

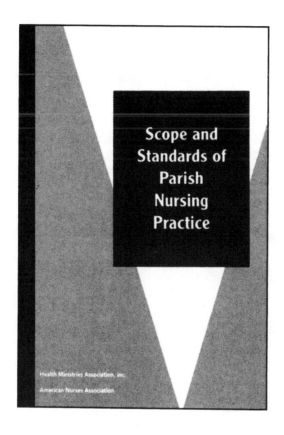

CONTENTS

INTRODUCTION

Parish nursing is a unique, specialized practice of professional nursing that focuses on the promotion of health within the context of the values, beliefs, and practices of a faith community, such as a church, synagogue, or mosque, and its mission and ministry to its members (families and individuals), and the community it serves.

Health is viewed as not only the absence of disease, but also as a sense of physical, social, psychological, and spiritual well-being and a sense of being in harmony with self, others, the environment, and God. Healing is the process of integrating the body, mind, and spirit to create wholeness, health, and a sense of well-being, even when curing may not occur.

Professional nursing is rooted in these concepts of health and healing. Parish nursing promotes health and healing within faith communities. With the recognition that most illnesses and premature deaths are a result of life-style choices about diet, exercise, substance abuse, violence, and risk-taking behaviors, parish nursing integrates current medical and behavioral knowledge with the beliefs and practices of a faith community to promote health as wholeness and to prevent or minimize illness.

The members of a profession are responsible for defining the scope and competent standards of practice for the profession that set it apart from other professions. The American Nurses Association (ANA) published the generic *Standards of Clinical Nursing Practice* in 1991. According to this document, "[s]tandards are authoritative statements by which the nursing profession describes the responsibilities for which its practitioners are accountable. Consequently, standards reflect the values and priorities of the profession. Standards provide direction for professional nursing practice and a framework for the evaluation of practice. . . . [S]tandards also define the nursing profession's accountability to the public and the client outcomes for which nurses are responsible. . . . *Standards of Clinical Nursing Practice* is generic in nature and applies to all registered nurses engaged in clinical practice, regardless of clinical specialty, practice setting, or educational preparation. A professional nursing organization has a responsibility to its membership and the public it serves to develop standards of practice." (ANA 1991, 1)

SCOPE OF PARISH NURSING PRACTICE

The *Standards of Clinical Nursing Practice* (ANA 1991) describes a competent level of nursing care and professional performance common to all nurses engaged in clinical practice. A nursing specialty builds upon the generic scope and standards of practice and further delineates the unique scope and standards of practice of the specialty. The scope and standards of practice of a specialty are developed for the purpose of guiding the professional practice of its practitioners and defining the specialty's accountability to the public it serves.

The purpose of this document, *Scope and Standards of Parish Nursing Practice*, is to describe the evolving speciality of parish nursing and to provide parish nurses, the nursing profession, other health care providers, employers, insurers, and their clients with the unique scope and competent standards of care and professional performance expected of a parish nurse. The development of standards of practice for parish nursing reflects the commitment of the Health Ministries Association, Inc., to promoting parish nursing as a specialized practice of nursing and of health ministry. The Health Ministries Association, Inc., is a professional organization representing parish nurses and other health ministers. The *Scope and Standards of Parish Nursing Practice* addresses the independent practice of professional nursing, as defined by the jurisdiction's nursing practice act, in health promotion within the context of the client's values, beliefs, and faith practices. The client focus of a parish nurse is the faith community, including its family and individual members and the community it serves.

Like the independent practice of nursing, parish nursing promotes health and healing by empowering the client system (faith community, family, or individual) to incorporate health and healing practices from its faith perspective to achieve desired outcomes. The scope and standards of parish nursing practice set forth in this document reflect current parish nursing practice, client health promotion needs, professional standards, and the legal scope of professional nursing practice. They are dynamic in nature and subject to testing and change.

Professional nurses may also be employed by faith communities to practice the dependent functions of nursing as defined by the nursing practice act of the jurisdiction in which practiced. However, the dependent functions of practice would not be considered within the scope of parish nursing practice as defined and described in this document. Nurses practicing the dependent functions of nursing must meet the legal criteria set forth in the jurisdiction's nursing practice act, must practice according to the generic professional standards of practice (ANA 1991), and must practice according to relevant specialty standards of practice, such as the standards for advanced nursing practice (ANA 1996).

The *Standards of Clinical Nursing Practice* (ANA 1991) recognizes that nursing care must be individualized to meet the unique needs and situation of a particular client, such as a faith community. "The nurse also must respect the client's goals and preferences in developing and implementing a plan of care. Given that one of the nurse's primary responsibilities is client education, nurses must provide clients with appropriate information to make informed decisions regarding their health care and treatment, including health promotion and prevention of disease. However, it is recognized that some state regulations or institutional policies and procedures may prohibit full disclosure of information to clients or may require reporting of confidential information" (ANA 1991, 4).

The *Scope and Standards of Parish Nursing Practice* presents standards of care and standards of professional performance and is based on the *Standards of Clinical Nursing Practice* (ANA 1991). The standards of care describe a competent level of parish nursing care as demonstrated by the nursing process: assessment, diagnosis, outcome identification, planning, implementation, and evaluation. Standards of care delineate care that is provided to all clients of parish nursing services and should take into account cultural, racial, ethnic, and world view diversity. Standards of professional performance describe a competent level of behavior in the parish nursing role: quality of care, performance appraisal, education, collegiality, ethics, collaboration, research, and resource utilization.

GLOSSARY

Assessment—A systematic, dynamic process of collecting and analyzing data for the purpose of identifying and planning for unmet actual, perceived, or potential psycho-social, physical, and spiritual health outcomes.

Client—A human system (faith community, family, individual) and its environment, viewed as an integrated whole for which the parish nurse provides specific health promotion services.

Criteria—Key indicators of competent parish nursing practice that allow the standard to be measured. Criteria reflect current professional standards and parish nursing practice. Criteria are revised periodically to remain current with the evolving knowledge and practice of parish nursing.

Diagnosis—A clinical judgment about the client's health status based on data obtained by assessing the client's response to actual, perceived, or potential health concerns or needs. The diagnosis is used to identify desired outcomes, establish priorities, and develop a plan of action with the client.

Documentation—The recording of the assessment, plan of care, interventions, and evaluation of outcomes in a retrievable format for the client in order to facilitate continuity in meeting desired health outcomes.

Employee—A person, such as a parish nurse, whose services are engaged by another person or organization (employer), such as a faith community, who provides parameters for actions for which the employer may be held legally accountable. An employee may or may not receive monetary compensation.

Evaluation—The process of determining the outcomes achieved, the effectiveness of the plan, and the satisfaction of the client with those outcomes, for the purpose of modifying the plan.

Faith community—An organization of families and individuals who share common values, beliefs, religious doctrine, and faith practices that influence their lives, such as a church, synagogue, or mosque, and that functions as a client system, a focus for parish nursing.

Healing—The process of integrating the body, mind, and spirit to achieve wholeness, health, and a sense of well-being, even when the curing of disease may not occur.

Health—Wholeness, salvation, shalom. The integration of the physical, psychological, social, and spiritual aspects of the client system and harmony with self, others, the environment, and God.

Health care providers—Individuals, agencies, or institutions having expertise in promoting health as wholeness, including faith communities.

Health care professionals—Health care providers (such as nurses, doctors, psychologists, social workers, clergy, etc.) who are legally and professionally authorized to provide prescribed health services in the jurisdictions in which they practice.

Health ministry—The promotion of health and healing as part of the mission and ministry of a faith community to its members and the community it serves.

Health promotion—Activities and interventions that client systems undertake to achieve desired health outcomes. Health promotion outcomes may be primary, the prevention of disease and injury; secondary, the early detection and appropriate intervention in illness/brokenness; or tertiary, the promotion of wholeness and sense of well-being when curing may not occur.

Illness—The experience of brokenness; dis-integration of body, mind, spirit; and dis-harmony with others, the environment, and God.

Implementation—The carrying out of a plan of action by providing the information, skills, motivation, and resources necessary to empower the client system to achieve desired health outcomes.

Outcomes—The measurable changes in health status as a result of the implementation of the health promotion plan.

Parish nurse—The most common title given to a registered professional nurse who serves as a member of the ministry staff of a faith community to promote health as wholeness of the faith community, its family and individual members, and the community it serves through the independent practice of nursing as defined by the nurse practice act in the jurisdiction in which he or she practices and the standards of practice set forth in this document.

Plan of care—The health promotion plan with the actions to be taken to achieve mutually identified health outcomes.

Self-care—Actions a client (faith community, family, individual) would take to attain desired health outcomes if they had the knowledge, skills, ability, resources, and motivation.

Standards—Authoritative statements that reflect the values held by the profession and the specialized area of practice and that set the level of competent care and professional performance for which its practitioners are held accountable.

STANDARDS OF CARE

Standard I.   Assessment

The parish nurse collects client health data.

Rationale

Data collection is essential to a realistic assessment of client health. Data are systematically obtained, validated, and recorded in a retrievable format in order for the parish nurse and the client to develop a realistic, effective plan for health promotion.

Measurement Criteria

1. The parish nurse systematically collects data that are appropriate, comprehensive, and accurate.

2. The amount, type/areas, and priority of data collection are determined by the client and the mutually identified desired health outcomes.

3. The parish nurse collaborates with others to collect data related to the health of the faith community, its families and individual members, and the community it serves.

4. Data may include but are not limited to the following:
    *   Demographic data about the various client systems
    *   Developmental status: mental and emotional, psychosocial, spiritual, and physical development
    *   Responses to health and illness
    *   Client system's functional status: organization (and function), ability to accomplish mission and goals, self-care abilities to achieve desired health outcomes
    *   Spiritual status: meaning and purpose, hope, energy, faith beliefs and practices
    *   Psychological: cognitive and emotional function, coping patterns

- Social conditions and factors influencing health: social support structure and function, communication skills, resources
- Environmental factors influencing health: physical, cultural, legal, political, economic
- Health-promoting and health-compromising behaviors
- Health history and patterns of illness
- Client expectations and sense of responsibility for care of self and others
- Accessible and available services and resources.

5. A variety of methods, tools, and sources are used to collect data.

6. Relevant data are recorded in a standardized, systematic, and concise form, retrievable by the client for use in self-care and in communication with health care providers.

7. The assessment process is ongoing.

8. Collected data are used to formulate diagnoses.

Standard II.   Diagnosis

The parish nurse analyzes collected data about the client to determine the diagnosis.

Rationale

The basis for the plan of care is the diagnosis. Diagnoses guide the mutual planning of primary, secondary, and tertiary health promotion interventions. They reflect the client's self-care abilities and deficits in achieving wholeness and are derived from nursing, theological, medical, sociological, and psychological theories and knowledge.

Measurement Criteria

1. Diagnoses identify actual, perceived, or potential threats to health/wholeness.

2. Diagnoses are holistic and are based on generally accepted classification systems.

3. Diagnoses and risk factors are validated with the client and other health care providers when appropriate.

4. Diagnoses are recorded in a manner that facilitates the client's achievement of the desired outcomes.

Standard III. Outcome Identification

The parish nurse, with the client, identifies expected outcomes specific to the client's desired health outcomes.

Rationale

The parish nurse assists clients in setting priorities and identifying realistic, achievable health outcomes congruent with their values, beliefs, and faith practices. Outcomes focus on achieving wholeness.

Measurement Criteria

1. Expected outcomes are derived from the diagnoses.

2. Expected outcomes are measurable goals developed for and with the client.

3. Expected outcomes are focused on the promotion of health as wholeness even in the presence of illness and brokenness.

4. Expected outcomes are realistic and achievable on the basis of the client's knowledge, skills, ability, resources, and motivation.

Standard IV. Planning

The parish nurse assists the client in developing a plan for health promotion and other interventions that empowers the client to achieve desired health outcomes. The plan identifies the self-care activities to be done by the client, the interdependence with other systems, the interventions to be performed by the parish nurse, and the collaboration with and referral to other health care professionals and providers on the basis of the expected outcomes.

Rationale

The plan of care logically guides client self-care actions and parish nursing interventions to facilitate achievement of the mutually desired outcomes. Each plan incorporates the client's values, faith beliefs, and practices.

Measurement Criteria

1. The health promotion plan is mutually developed with the client.

2. The plan identifies a sequence of actions for achieving measurable outcomes.

3. The plan uses effective actions and interventions based on relevant nursing and scientific knowledge and the faith beliefs and practices of the client.

4. The plan proposes contingency actions for changes in the client's health status, self-care abilities, or outcomes.

Standard V. Implementation

The parish nurse assists the client in implementing the interventions identified in the health promotion plan.

Rationale

The parish nurse empowers the client to implement the plan in collaboration with the parish nurse, other health ministers, and other health care providers in order to facilitate the promotion of the client's health. The parish nurse's interventions are within the independent scope of practice of nursing as defined by the jurisdiction in which he or she is practicing and within the nurse's knowledge and skill. Interventions are competent and based on acceptable health care practices.

Measurement Criteria

1. Interventions are based on the mutually developed plan.

2. Interventions integrate the client's values, faith beliefs, and practices.

3. Intervention empowers the client to use self-care abilities to
   - Promote wholeness
   - Prevent illness
   - Cope with changes in health status.

4. Interventions are within the legal, professional, and employer's defined scope of practice and may include—
   - Enhancing and monitoring self-care and care-giving abilities
   - Health teaching
   - Primary, secondary, and tertiary health promotion programs
   - Health counseling
   - Collaboration with and referral to appropriate health care providers to ensure continuity of care
   - Information and assistance in obtaining resources
   - Advocacy for services and policies that affect client health.

5. Interventions reflect consideration of the client's uniqueness, integrity, and autonomy.

6. Interventions are recorded in a standardized and concise manner to provide the client and other care providers with the necessary documentation for continuity of care.

Standard VI. Evaluation

The parish nurse continually evaluates client responses to interventions in order to determine the progress made toward desired outcomes.

Rationale

Parish nursing practice is a dynamic process. The effectiveness of parish nursing depends on the continual reassessment of the client's health status and appropriate revisions of the plan until mutually established outcomes are achieved.

Measurement Criteria

1. Evaluation is systematic and ongoing.

2. The effectiveness of interventions is evaluated in relation to outcome criteria.

3. Observations are validated with the client and other health care providers.

4. Revision of the health promotion plan and its priorities, desired outcomes, and interventions is conducted in collaboration with the client and is based on the evaluation of outcomes.

STANDARDS OF PROFESSIONAL PERFORMANCE

Standard I. Quality of Care

The parish nurse systematically participates in evaluation of the quality and effectiveness of his or her parish nursing practice.

Rationale

Parish nursing is an evolving specialty in nursing and has an expanding body of knowledge and research that provides the parish nurse with the information necessary for improving the quality and effectiveness of the practice.

Measurement Criteria

1. The parish nurse initiates and participates in self-evaluation and evaluation of the overall health ministry program in order to acknowledge nursing actions and improve the quality of services provided.

2. The parish nurse participates in peer and interdisciplinary groups whose members may include clergy, other health ministers, and clients who review and evaluate the effectiveness of the parish nursing practice as a part of a health ministry of a faith community by—
   - Identifying aspects of practice that are important for quality monitoring, such as interpreting health as wholeness, the integration of spiritual care in health promotion, health education, health counseling, advocacy, promotion of self-care, and care giving
   - Monitoring the appropriateness and comprehensiveness of the process of care components (assessment, diagnosis, outcome identification, planning, implementation, and evaluation)
   - Analyzing statistical data for trends in client populations, recurring and emerging health needs and concerns, and areas requiring additional resources

- Obtaining client feedback on satisfaction with outcomes
- Determining effectiveness in the use of time, energy, and resources to achieve outcomes
- Developing policies and procedures to improve the parish nursing practice.

3. The parish nurse assumes responsibility for monitoring the quality of care based on education, experience, and the practice environment.

4. The parish nurse incorporates appropriate changes for improving the quality of care and client outcomes as suggested by the evaluation processes.

Standard II. Performance Appraisal

The parish nurse evaluates his or her own nursing practice in relation to professional standards, relevant statutes, and regulations.

Rationale

The parish nurse is accountable to all clients, the profession, and the public for providing competent nursing care and for practicing according to the standards established by the specialty, the profession, and regulatory bodies.

Measurement Criteria

1. The parish nurse systematically engages in performance appraisal of his or her own parish nursing practice and role performance.

2. The parish nurse invites appraisal of his or her performance as a parish nurse by peers and administrative super-

visors, such as the clergy and administrative council, and incorporates these appraisals into his or her personal and professional development plans.

3. The parish nurse encourages and facilitates peer review activities for him- or herself and other parish nurses.

Standard III. Education

The parish nurse acquires and maintains current knowledge in nursing practice and health promotion.

Rationale

The clients of a parish nurse represent the total life span of three client levels: the faith community and its families and individuals. Each client presents unique physical, psycho-social, and spiritual developmental stages; risks to health; and cultural and socioeconomic diversity. Hence, the parish nurse must continually update his or her knowledge of nursing science, public health, and medicine, in addition to acquiring knowledge in theology, psychology, and sociology, in order to enhance the practice of parish nursing. Formal education, continuing education, self-study, and experiential learning are all means for professional growth.

Measurement Criteria

1. The parish nurse seeks out educational activities in order to improve clinical knowledge and skills, enhance role performance, and increase his or her level of competency as a parish nurse.

2. The parish nurse acquires the knowledge and skills necessary to practice as a competent parish nurse in areas of deficit identified by this document, self-assessment, quality-of-care evaluations, and performance appraisals.

Standard IV. Collegiality

The parish nurse contributes to the professional development of peers, colleagues, and other health ministers.

Rationale

The parish nurse is responsible for promoting the health promotion abilities of others through appropriate informal and formal teaching and collaboration with colleagues.

Measurement Criteria

1. The parish nurse shares knowledge and skills with others.

2. The parish nurse creates an environment conducive to the clinical education of nurses and other health care providers.

3. The parish nurse participates in the development of educational programs for health care providers and health ministers that focus on the concept of health and healing from a faith perspective.

Standard V. Ethics

The parish nurse's decisions and actions reflect and are guided by client, personal, and professional ethical considerations.

Rationale

The parish nurse is responsible for providing health promotion services to promote the client's desired health outcomes. With the inevitable conflicts among client, societal, professional, and personal beliefs and values, the parish nurse must have knowledge of these beliefs and values and make ethical decisions in a systematic manner that respects client values and belief systems and achieves the best possible outcome. Ethical concerns in parish nursing include the principles of client autonomy, the right of self-determination in health care decisions and confidentiality; beneficence/nonmaleficence, the obligation to do good and not to do harm; and justice, the distribution of limited resources (including time, energy, and fiscal and material resources). In addition, parish nurses ought to consider the virtue ethics, such as caring, forgiveness, and compassion, in their decision making.

Measurement Criteria

1. The parish nurse's practice is guided by the *Code for Nurses with Interpretive Statements* (ANA 1985).

2. The parish nurse maintains a professional and therapeutic relationship with the client at all times.

3. The parish nurse respects the decisions of the client without being judgmental and delivers nondiscriminatory health promotion services.

4. The parish nurse identifies real and potential ethical conflicts and seeks the facts and resources to assist him- or herself and clients in making ethical decisions.

5. The parish nurse is an advocate for the client's right to self-determination and for support in the carrying out of health care decisions that reflect the client's beliefs, values, and faith practices.

6. The parish nurse reports unethical and illegal activities to the appropriate authorities.

7. The parish nurse educates clients about their rights and responsibilities in making informed health care decisions.

8. The parish nurse does not abandon a client when there is unresolved conflict between the client's and the nurse's values, but refers to appropriate resources.

9. The parish nurse maintains confidentiality at all times.

Standard VI. Collaboration

The parish nurse collaborates with the client system, other health ministers, health care providers, and community agencies in promoting client health.

Rationale

The unique breadth and depth of parish nursing require extensive use of all resources necessary to promote health and healing for all client systems—faith community, family, and individual. Through the use of a collaborative practice model, parish nurses are best able to promote client health. A holistic approach to health promotion requires the special abilities and resources of all health care providers and health care professionals who share a commitment to promoting health and healing.

Measurement Criteria

1. The parish nurse collaborates with the client, other health ministers, and other health care providers in decision making about the client's health promotion plan, interventions, and desired outcomes.

2. The parish nurse respects, appreciates, and encourages the contributions of clients, health ministers, health care professionals, and providers in promoting the role of the faith community in health and healing.

3. The parish nurse articulates the role and practice of parish nursing to clients and other health care providers.

4. The parish nurse consults with and refers to other health care providers as needed and integrates their expertise into the health promotion plan.

Standard VII. Research

The parish nurse uses research findings in practice.

Rationale

The parish nurse is responsible for using current research findings and contributing to the improvement of his or her own current and future parish nursing practice through research, on the basis of his or her level of education and practice environment.

Measurement Criteria

1. The parish nurse uses health promotion interventions substantiated by research and based on effectiveness data.

2. The parish nurse participates in research to validate and improve the parish nursing practice and health ministry. On the basis of the level of education and practice setting, research activities may include—
    *   Identifying practices and problems for research
    *   Collecting data for research
    *   Conducting and disseminating research findings
    *   Incorporating research into the faith community's health ministry and parish nursing policies and procedures
    *   Providing significant research findings to clients, peers, and other health promoters.

Standard VIII. Resource Utilization

The parish nurse considers the effectiveness measures of appropriateness, accessibility, acceptability, and affordability of resources in the development and implementation of health promotion programs for clients.

Rationale

Clients are entitled to a parish nursing practice that is safe and effective. The parish nurse must facilitate a health ministry that maximizes resources to achieve the desired health outcomes for all clients.

Measurement Criteria

1. The parish nurse evaluates the effective use of resources (such as time, energy, and fiscal and material resources) to achieve desired client outcomes as measured by appropriateness, accessibility, acceptability, and affordability.

2. The parish nurse assists clients in choosing and obtaining resources that are safe and effective.

3. The parish nurse uses the client's beliefs, values, and faith practices to guide decisions in the allocation of scarce resources.

REFERENCES

American Nurses Association. 1996. *Scope and Standards of Advanced Practice Registered Nursing.* Washington, DC: American Nurses Association.

American Nurses Association. 1991. *Standards of Clinical Nursing Practice.* Washington, DC: American Nurses Association.

American Nurses Association. 1985. *Code for Nurses with Interpretive Statements.* Washington, DC: American Nurses Association.

ACKNOWLEDGMENTS

This document was developed by the Practice and Education Committee of the Health Ministries Association, Inc. The Board of Directors gratefully acknowledges the contribution of the parish nurse members who reviewed and submitted comments and recommendations during its development.

Practice and Education Committee

Wendy RuthStiver, MA, BSN, RN, Chairperson, Monrovia, CA
Norma R. Small, PhD, CRNP, Standards of Practice Advisor, Johnstown, PA
Mary Chase-Zoilek, PhD, RN, Chicago, IL
The Rev. Jean Denton, RN, Deacon, Indianapolis, IN
Lou-Anne Keith, MSN, RN, Anaheim, CA

Adopted by the Board of Directors September 23, 1996.
Revised January 1998.

Acknowledged by the American Nurses Association, Congress of Nursing Practice, February 1998.

Library of Congress Cataloging-in-Publication Data

Scope and standards of parish nursing practice / Health Ministries
    Association, American Nurses Association ; [developed by the
    Practice and Education Committee of the Health Ministries
    Association].
        p.   cm.
    Includes bibliographical references.
    1. Nursing—Religious aspects—Standards—United States.
    I. Health Ministries Association. Practice and Education Committee.
    II. American Nurses Association
RT85.2.S37   1998
610.73—dc21   98-23242
                                                          CIP

Published by   Health Ministries Association, Inc.
American Nurses Publishing   1930 Cedar Street
600 Maryland Avenue, SW   Ramona, CA 92065
Suite 100 West
Washington, DC 20024-2571

First printing June 1998. Second printing 1998. Third printing
January 2002. Fourth printing October 2002.
9806ST   3M   10/02R

INDEX

A year in brackets [1998] indicates an entry from *Scope and Standards of Parish Nursing Practice* (1998), reproduced in Appendix A.

A
Advanced practice faith community nursing
assessment, 11
collaboration, 28
collegiality, 27
consultation, 20
coordination of care, 18
defined, 6, 35
diagnosis, 12
education, 25
ethics, 29
evaluation, 22
health teaching and health promotion, 19
implementation, 17–21
leadership, 32–33
outcomes identification, 13–14
planning, 15–16
prescriptive authority and treatment, 21
professional practice evaluation, 26
quality of practice, 23–24
research, 30
resource utilization, 31
roles, 6, 7
See also Faith community nursing; Generalist faith community nursing
Advocacy for patients and families, 1, 6
coordination of care and, 18
ethics and, 29
[1998] 61
implementation and, [1998] 55
quality of care and, [1998] 57

Age-appropriate care. *See* Cultural competence
American Nurses Association (ANA), *v, vi*
[1998] 45
Code of Ethics with Interpretive Statements, v, 1, 10
Nursing: Scope and Standards of Practice, vi, 1, 3, 10
Nursing's Social Policy Statement, v, 1, 10
Standards of Clinical Nursing Practice, [1998] 45, 46, 47
Analysis. *See* Critical thinking, analysis, and synthesis
Assessment, *vii,* 3
[1998] 47
defined, 35, [1998] 48
diagnosis and, 12
evaluation and, 22
[1998] 56
planning and, 16
prescriptive authority and treatment, 21
quality of care and, [1998] 57
standard of practice, 11
[1998] 51–52
tools, 3

B
Body of knowledge, 4, 8, 9
education and, 25
implementation and, 17
planning and, [1998] 54
prescriptive authority and treatment, 21

quality of care and, [1998] 57
research and, 30

C

Care recipient. *See* Patient
Care standards. *See* Standards of
  practice
Caregiver (defined), 35
Case management. *See* Coordination
  of care
Certification and credentialing, 1, 5
Client (defined), [1998] 48
  See also Faith Community;
    Family; Patient
Clinical Nurse Specialist (CNS), 6, 35
Clinical settings. *See* Practice settings
Code of ethics (defined), 35
Code of Ethics for Nurses with
  Interpretive Statements, v, 1, 10, 29
  [1998] 61
  See also Ethics
Collaboration, *viii,* 4, 7, 8, 9
  [1998] 47
  collegiality and, [1998] 60
  evaluation and, [1998] 56
  implementation and, 17
    [1998] 55
  outcomes identification and, 13
  planning and, [1998] 54
  standard of professional
    performance, 28
    [1998] 62
  See also Healthcare providers;
    Interdisciplinary health care;
    Referrals
Collegiality, *viii,* 8
  [1998] 47
  diagnosis and, 12
  implementation and, 17
  professional practice evaluation
    and, 26

[1998] 58, 59
quality of care and, [1998] 57
standard of professional
  performance, 27
  [1998] 60
Communication, 8
  assessment and, [1998] 52
  collaboration and, 28
  collegiality and, 27
    [1998] 60
  evaluation and, 22
  leadership and, 33
  planning and, 15
  professional practice evaluation
    and, 26
  research and, 30
    [1998] 63
Community health care, 1, 4, 8
  [1998] 45
  assessment and, [1998] 51
  collaboration and, [1998] 62
  implementation and, 17
Compensation, 10
Competence assessment. *See*
  Certification and credentialing
Confidentiality, [1998] 47
  assessment and, 11
  coordination of care and, 18
  See also Ethics
Congregational nurse, 2
  See also Faith community
    nursing
Consultation, *vii,* 1, 6
  standard of practice, 20
Continuity of care
  collaboration and, 28
  coordination of care and, 18
  defined, 35
  outcomes identification and, 13,
    14
  planning and, 15

implementation and, [1998] 55
outcomes identification and, 13
planning and, 16
    [1998] 54
professional practice evaluation
    and, 26
resource utilization and, [1998]
    64
See also Spiritual health

D
Data (defined), 35
Data collection, 10
    assessment and, 11
        [1998] 51
    diagnosis and, [1998] 52
    quality of practice and, 23
    research and, 30
        [1998] 63
Deacon, 7
    See also Advanced practice faith
    community nursing
Decision-making, [1998] 47
    collaboration and, 28
        [1998] 62
    consultation and, 20
    ethics and, 29
        [1998] 60, 61
    leadership and, 33
    planning and, 16
    research and, 30
    resource utilization and, [1998]
    64
Diagnosis, *vii*, 3
    [1998] 47
    assessment and, 11
        [1998] 52
    defined, 35
        [1998] 48
    evaluation and, 22
    outcomes identification and, 13
        [1998] 53

planning and, 15, 16
prescriptive authority and
    treatment, 21
quality of care and, [1998] 57
standard of practice, 12
    [1998] 52–53
Disease (defined), 35
Documentation
    assessment and, 11
        [1998] 51, 52
    collaboration and, 28
    coordination of care and, 18
    defined, 36
        [1998] 48
    diagnosis and, 12
    education and, 25
    evaluation and, 22
    implementation and, 17
        [1998] 56
    outcomes identification and, 13
    quality of practice and, 23

E
Economic issues. *See* Cost control
Education of patients and families, 1,
    3, 4, 8
    [1998] 47, 55
    See also Family; Health teaching
        and health promotion; Patient
Education of faith community
    nurses, *viii*, 1, 4, 8
    [1998] 47
    collegiality and, 27
        [1998] 60
    leadership and, 32
    quality of care and, [1998] 58
    requirements, 5, 6, 9
    research and, 30
        [1998] 63
    standard of professional
    performance, 25
        [1998] 59

evaluation and, 22
outcomes identification and, 13
See also Education of patients
and families; Patient
Financial issues. *See* Cost control

G
Generalist faith community nursing, 5
assessment, 11
[1998] 51–52
collaboration, 28
[1998] 62
collegiality, 27
[1998] 60
consultation, 20
coordination of care, 18
diagnosis, 12
[1998] 52–53
education, 25
[1998] 59
ethics, 29
[1998] 60–61
evaluation, 22
[1998] 56
health teaching and health
promotion, 19
implementation, 17–21
[1998] 54–56
leadership, 32
outcomes identification, 13
[1998] 53
planning, 15–16
[1998] 54
prescriptive authority and
treatment, 21
professional practice evaluation,
26
[1998] 58–59
quality of practice, 23–24
[1998] 57–58
research, 30

[1998] 63
resource utilization, 31
[1998] 63–64
roles, 5–6, 8
See also Advanced practice faith
community nursing; Faith
community nursing
Group (defined), 36
Guidelines
defined, 37
outcomes identification and, 14
leadership and, 33
professional practice evaluation
and, 26
quality of practice and, 23

H
Healing (defined), 3, 37
[1998] 45, 49
Health (defined), 2, 37
[1998] 45, 49
See also Spiritual health;
Wholistic health
Health Ministries Association (HMA),
vi, 8
[1998] 46
Health ministry (defined), 37
[1998] 49
Health ministry nurse, 2
See also Faith community
nursing
Health teaching and health
promotion, *vii,* 7
[1998] 45, 46, 47
assessment and, [1998] 51, 52
collaboration and, [1998] 62
collegiality and, [1998] 60
defined, 37
[1998] 49
diagnosis and, [1998] 52
education and, [1998] 59

ethics and, [1998] 60, 61
implementation and, 17
  [1998] 54, 55
outcomes identification and,
  [1998] 53
planning and, 15
  [1998] 54
quality of care and, [1998] 57
standard of practice, 19
research and, [1998] 63
resource utilization and, [1998]
  63
Health and wellness nurse, 2
  See also Faith community
    nursing
Healthcare policy
  quality of practice and, 23
    [1998] 58
  research and, 30
    [1998] 63
Healthcare professionals (defined),
  [1998] 49
Healthcare providers, 1, 6, 8
  [1998] 46
  assessment and, 11
    [1998] 52
  collaboration and, 28
    [1998] 62
  collegiality and, 27
    [1998] 60
  coordination of care and, 18
  defined, 37
    [1998] 49
  diagnosis and, 12
    [1998] 53
  evaluation and, 22
    [1998] 56
  implementation and, [1998] 55
  leadership and, 32
  outcomes identification and, 13
  planning and, [1998] 54

quality of practice and, 23
research and, [1998] 63
See also Collaboration;
  Interdisciplinary health care
Healthcare team. See Collaboration;
  Interdisciplinary health care
Healthy People 2010, 9
Holistic. See Wholistic health
Human resources. See Professional
  development

I
Illness (defined), 37
  [1998] 49
Implementation, vii, 6
  [1998] 47
  coordination of care and, 18
  defined, 37
    [1998] 50
  evaluation and, 22
  planning and, 15
  quality of practice and, 23
    [1998] 57
  resource utilization and, [1998]
    63
  standard of practice, 17–21
    [1998] 54–56
Information. See Data collection
Intentional care, 3, 5
Interdisciplinary health care, 5, 6, 7, 8, 9
  collaboration and, 28
  collegiality and, 27
  coordination of care and, 18
  defined, 37
  ethics and, 29
  implementation and, 17
  leadership and, 33
  planning and, 15
  quality of practice and, 23
  research and, 30
  resource utilization and, 31

evaluation and, 22
  [1998] 56
implementation and, 17
leadership and, 33
planning and, 15
  [1998] 54
quality of practice and, 23
resource utilization and, 31
See also Evaluation; Outcomes
  identification

P

Parents. See Family
Parish nursing, 2
  [1998] 43–67
  defined, [1998] 45, 50
  See also Faith community
    nursing
Pastoral Associate, 7
  See also Advanced practice faith
    community nursing
Pastoral care (defined), 38
Patient, 3–4, 7
  [1998] 45, 47
  assessment and, 11
    [1998] 51
  collaboration and, 28
    [1998] 62
  consultation and, 20
  defined, 1, 38
  diagnosis and, 12
    [1998] 53
  education and, [1998] 59
  ethics and, 29
    [1998] 61
  evaluation and, 22
    [1998] 56
  outcomes identification and, 13, 14
    [1998] 53
  planning and, 15
    [1998] 54

professional practice evaluation
  and, 26
quality of care and, [1998] 57, 58
resource utilization and, 31
  [1998] 64
rights, 29
  [1998] 61
See also Education of patients
  and families; Family
Peer review (defined), 38
Performance appraisal, [1998] 47
  standard of professional
performance, [1998] 58–59
  See also Professional practice
    evaluation
Pharmacologic agents. See
  Prescriptive authority
Plan of care (defined), [1998] 50
Planning, vii, 7
  [1998] 47
  assessment and, [1998] 51
  collaboration and, 28
    [1998] 62
  collegiality and, 27
  consultation and, 20
  coordination of care and, 18
  defined, 38
  diagnosis and, [1998] 52
  evaluation and, 22
    [1998] 56
  implementation and, 17
    [1998] 54, 55
  leadership and, 32
  outcomes identification and, 13
  quality of care and, [1998] 57
  resource utilization and, 31
  standard of practice, 15–16
    [1998] 54
Policy. See Healthcare policy
Practice environment, 7
  collegiality and, 27

[1998] 60
coordination of care and, 18
leadership and, 32
quality of practice and, 24
[1998] 58
research and, [1998] 63
Practice settings, 1, 7
[1998] 45, 46
Preceptors. *See* Mentoring
Prescriptive authority and treatment,
vii
standard of practice, 21
Privacy. *See* Confidentiality
Process. *See* Nursing process
Professional development, 1, 8
collegiality and, 27
[1998] 60
education and, 25
[1998] 59
leadership and, 32
professional practice evaluation
and, 26
[1998] 59
research and, 25
See also Education; Leadership
Professional organizations, 32
Professional performance. *See*
Standards of professional
performance
Professional practice evaluation, *viii*
collegiality and, 27
education and, [1998] 59
health teaching and health
promotion, 19
research and, [1998] 57
standard of professional
performance, 26

Q
Quality of care, [1998] 47
defined, 38
education and, [1998] 59

standard of professional
performance, [1998] 57–58
See also Quality of practice
Quality of life, 9, 14
Quality of practice, *viii*, 6
evaluation and, 22
resource utilization and, 31
standard of professional
performance, 23–24

R
Recipient of care. *See* Patient
Referrals, 1
planning and, [1998] 54
prescriptive authority and
treatment, 21
See also Collaboration;
Coordination of care
Regulatory issues. *See* Laws, statutes,
and regulations
Religious beliefs. *See* Spiritual health
Research, *viii*, 6, 8–9
[1998] 47
collaboration and, 28
education and, 25
planning and, 15, 16
quality of practice and, 24
[1998] 57
standard of professional
performance, 30
[1998] 63
See also Evidence-based practice
Resource utilization, *viii*, 1, 8
[1998] 47
assessment and, [1998] 52
collaboration and, 28
[1998] 62
coordination of care and, 18
ethics and, [1998] 61
health teaching and health
promotion, 19
implementation and, 17